REHABILITATION OF THE HAND AND UPPER EXTREMITY (EVERYTHING YOU MUST KNOW)

A Quick Practical complete Guide

Susan Skirven

Table of Contents

CHAPTER ONE 3

Introduction to Hand and Upper Extremity Rehabilitation 3

CHAPTER TWO 10

Knowing the Anatomy of the Hand and Upper Extremities 10

Common Conditions Affecting the Hand and Upper Extremity 19

CHAPTER THREE 26

The Rehabilitation Process 26

Techniques for Pain Management 30

CHAPTER FOUR 33

Treatment Techniques in Hand and Upper Extremity 33

Rehabilitation Modalities 41

CHAPTER FIVE 48

Therapeutic Interventions for Specific Conditions 48

Psychological Considerations in Rehabilitation 61

CHAPTER SIX 68

Recovery and Long-Term Management 68

Preventing Re-injury 75

THE END 83

CHAPTER ONE
Introduction to Hand and Upper Extremity Rehabilitation

Physical therapy's hand and upper extremity rehabilitation is a specialty that focuses on regaining strength, function, and mobility in the hands, wrists, arms, elbows, and shoulders. For those who have had surgeries, injuries, or illnesses impacting these areas, this kind of rehabilitation is crucial.

A quick overview of hand and upper extremity rehabilitation is provided here:

Assessment and Evaluation: A licensed therapist will usually conduct a comprehensive assessment as the first step in the rehabilitation process. Range of motion, strength, coordination, sensibility, and functional abilities of the hand and upper extremities may all be assessed during this evaluation.

Goal Setting: The therapist works with the patient to set rehabilitation goals based on the results of the evaluation as well as the individual's unique requirements and objectives. These objectives could be to strengthen the grip, increase range of motion, lessen pain, or improve functional abilities for tasks relating to daily living and the workplace.

Treatment Planning: Following goal-setting, the therapist creates a personalized treatment plan based on the requirements of the patient. Therapeutic exercises, manual therapy methods, splinting, functional training, and heat, cold, ultrasound, or electrical stimulation are a few examples of treatment approaches.

Therapeutic activities: In the rehabilitation of the hands and upper extremities, therapeutic activities are essential. The aforementioned exercises are designed to enhance the affected area's muscle and joint strength, flexibility, endurance, and coordination. Proprioceptive exercises, resistance training, stretching techniques, and neuromuscular reeducation are a few examples.

Manual Therapy: To increase tissue healing, lessen discomfort, and improve joint mobility, manual therapy techniques like massage and soft tissue mobilization are frequently utilized. These manual methods can be used to treat adhesions, stiffness, and tightness in the hand and upper extremity muscles, ligaments, and joints.

Orthotics and Splinting: During the healing phase, splints and orthotic devices may be recommended to support and shield the hand and upper extremities. These tools can support healthy alignment, lessen strain on damaged tissues, and enable useful movement patterns.

Education and Home Exercise Program: An integral part of the rehabilitation process for hands and upper extremities is patient education. In order to maximize rehabilitation and minimize the risk of re-injury, therapists train patients on appropriate body mechanics, ergonomics, activity moderation, and self-management techniques. Additionally, in order to continue their rehabilitation outside of therapy sessions, patients are usually provided a home workout routine.

Throughout the rehabilitation process, progress is regularly tracked, and treatment plans are modified as necessary in response to the patient's response to therapy. Therapists can monitor progress and make well-informed judgments about continued care by using outcome measures, functional assessments, and patient feedback.

Rehabilitation seeks to maximize healing, restore independence, and enhance quality of life for those with hand and upper extremity impairments and functional limits. These persons may have undergone operations, sustained injuries, or other disorders affecting these regions.

CHAPTER TWO
Knowing the Anatomy of the Hand and Upper Extremities

Comprehending the hand and upper extremity's anatomy is essential to understanding its movement and function. Let's examine each part in turn:

Bones:

There are multiple bones in the hand and upper extremities, including:

Shoulder Girdle: This comprises the scapula (shoulder blade) and clavicle (collarbone), which serve as attachment places for the muscles and upper arm.

Upper Arm: The long bone in the upper arm that joins the elbow joint to the shoulder is called the humerus.

Forearm: The radius and ulna are the two bones that make up the forearm. Pronation, or rotating the forearm palm down, and supination, or rotating the forearm palm up, are made possible by the way these bones articulate with one another at the elbow and wrist joints.

Eight carpal bones, organized in two rows, make up the wrist. These bones articulate with the hand's metacarpal bones and the forearm bones.

Hand: The hand is made up of fourteen phalanges, or finger bones, comprising two phalanges for the thumb and three phalanges for each finger. It also consists of five metacarpal bones, which comprise the palm.

Muscles:

Movement and function of the hand and upper extremities are facilitated by a multitude of muscles:

Shoulder Muscles: These muscles regulate mobility of the shoulder joint and include the deltoid, rotator cuff muscles (supraspinatus, infraspinatus, teres minor, and subscapularis), among others.

Arm Muscles: The elbow joint's flexion and extension are controlled by muscles like the triceps brachii and biceps brachii.

The flexor and extensor muscles in the forearm are responsible for controlling the movement of the wrist and fingers.

Hand Muscles: The hand's intrinsic and extrinsic muscles, which start in the forearm and extend into the hand, regulate the thumb, fingers, and grip strength.

Tendons and Ligaments:

Ligaments, which connect bones to provide support to joints, are fibrous bands of connective tissue. Fibrous cords called tendon connect muscles to bones and transfer the force produced by muscle contractions into motion.

Ligaments and tendons are essential for supporting joints and promoting movement in the hand and upper extremities. For instance, the hand's flexor and extensor tendons allow for the movement of the fingers and wrist, while ligaments support the stability of joints during different activities.

Anxiety:

Numerous nerves from the brachial plexus, a network of nerves made comprised of the spinal nerves of the cervical and thoracic regions, innervate the hand and upper extremities. Important nerves consist of:

The palm, thumb, index finger, middle finger, and half of the ring finger are all sensed by the medial nerve. Additionally, it innervates some of the muscles that move the thumb.

The little finger and a portion of the ring finger are supplied with feeling by the ulnar nerve. Additionally, it innervates the hand's fine motor muscles.

The radial nerve regulates the muscles that extend the wrist and fingers and provides feeling to the back of the hand.

Movement and Function:

The functions of the hand and upper extremities are numerous and include:

Holding and working with objects raising and transporting

Pulling and pushing

Reaching and stretching

turning and bending

Coordinated motions of muscles, tendons, ligaments, and nerves enable these movements, which provide dexterity, strength, and accuracy in a variety of daily activities, occupational activities, sports, and recreational pursuits. Humans are able to interact with their surroundings and carry out difficult activities with amazing agility and versatility due to the complex anatomy and physiology of the hand and upper extremity.

Common Conditions Affecting the Hand and Upper Extremity

Sprains, strains, and fractures:

Breaks or cracks in the hand, wrist, forearm, or upper arm are referred to as fractures. They may be brought on by falls, trauma, or ongoing stress.

Sprains: Sprains are caused by a tearing or stretching of the ligaments that attach bones to one another. They frequently affect the fingers or wrist.

Strains: Strains occur when muscles or tendons, which join muscles to bones, are torn or stretched. Overuse or abrupt motions might cause them to appear in the hand or forearm.

arthritic

Osteoarthritis: This degenerative joint disease can cause pain, stiffness, and a reduction in range of motion in the hand and finger joints.

Rheumatoid arthritis: An autoimmune disease that can cause inflammation, deformity, and impairment of function in a number of joints, including the hand and wrist.

Bursitis and tendinitis:

Inflammation of the tendons in the hand or wrist, frequently brought on by overuse or repeated motions, is known as tendinitis.

Bursitis: Inflammation of the bursae, which are fluid-filled sacs that cushion the joints; typically affects the elbow or shoulder.

Nerve Damage:

Peripheral nerve injuries: These can cause pain, weakness, numbness, or tingling. They can also be caused by trauma, compression, or stretching of the nerves in the hand or upper extremity.

Brachial Plexus Injuries: These injuries, which are frequently brought on by birthing trauma, accidents, or sports-related injuries, affect the network of nerves that regulate movement and feeling in the shoulder, arm, and hand.

Carpal Tunnel Syndrome:

compression of the median nerve causing pain, numbness, tingling, and weakness in the hand and fingers as it travels through the carpal tunnel in the wrist.

Finger Trigger:

a disorder where the fingers' tendons become inflamed or thickened, making it difficult to straighten the fingers and causing them to catch or lock in place.

Dupuytren's Tendinopathy:

a disorder where the fingers are drawn into a bent position and are difficult to straighten due to thickening and shortening of the connective tissue in the palm of the hand.

Amputation:

surgical excision of a limb—including the fingers, hands, or arms—because of an accident, an illness, or a medical condition like cancer or vascular disease.

Birthmarks:

Congenital hand anomalies, such as syndactyly or polydactyly, which include abnormal development of the fingers, thumbs, or hands, are examples of conditions that exist from birth.

These are but a handful of the numerous ailments that can impact the hand and upper limb. Depending on the severity and underlying cause, each ailment may require a different course of treatment, such as medication, physical therapy, bracing, splinting, injections, or surgery. To maximize results and maintain hand and upper extremity function, early diagnosis and treatments are essential.

CHAPTER THREE
The Rehabilitation Process

Of course! The following summarizes the hand and upper extremity rehabilitation process:

Stages of Recovery:

Acute Phase: This stage, which usually starts right away following an injury or surgery, is dedicated to protecting the wounded area, reducing swelling, and managing discomfort. Gentle mobilizations and passive range-of-motion exercises can be started to avoid stiffness and encourage early healing.

Subacute Phase: Restoring function, strength, and range of motion becomes more important as the healing process advances. To increase mobility, stability, and coordination, functional activities, manual treatment methods, and therapeutic exercises are progressively added.

Chronic Phase: The goal of this phase is to optimize independence, endurance, and function in day-to-day activities and functional tasks. To maximize long-term results and avoid re-injury, functional reintegration, activity-specific training, and advanced therapeutic exercises are prioritized.

The Value of Prompt Intervention

Promoting the best possible recovery and avoiding problems require early intervention. Early rehabilitation following surgery or injury can reduce pain, edema, and stiffness, avoid muscle atrophy, and promote a quicker return to normal function. Timely assessment and treatment of underlying impairments is another benefit of early intervention that can enhance results and lower the chance of long-term incapacity.

Establishing Expectations and Goals:

Establishing attainable objectives is crucial for directing the recovery process and inspiring the person. Objectives ought to be time-bound, relevant, measurable, achievable, and specific (SMART). Rehabilitation efforts are more likely to be in line with the patient's personal goals and way of life when meaningful goals are developed in partnership with them, based on their functional needs, priorities, and expectations.

Techniques for Pain Management

The rehabilitation process requires effective pain management, which may involve a mix of pharmacological and non-pharmacological interventions:

Medication: To reduce pain and inflammation, doctors may prescribe muscle relaxants, analgesics, and nonsteroidal anti-inflammatory medications (NSAIDs).

Therapeutic modalities: To lessen discomfort, edema, and muscular spasm, practitioners may employ ice packs, heat packs, ultrasounds, electrical stimulation, and laser therapy.

Manual therapy: Manual methods including massage, joint mobility, and soft tissue mobilization can help reduce pain, enhance circulation, and encourage tissue repair.

Activity Modification: Adaptive equipment or activity modifications can assist reduce pain and stop symptoms from getting worse while performing daily duties.

Education: Giving people knowledge on ergonomics, relaxation methods, pain management techniques, and self-care tactics helps them manage their pain more skillfully and improves their general wellbeing.

Effective pain management facilitates more seamless rehabilitation, enabling patients to engage fully in treatment and more comfortably and confidently reach their recovery objectives.

CHAPTER FOUR
Treatment Techniques in Hand and Upper Extremity

Several therapeutic approaches are used in hand and upper extremity rehabilitation to encourage healing and enhance function. Here are a few methods that are often employed:

Rehabilitative Exercise:

A crucial part of hand and upper extremity therapy is therapeutic exercise. Strength, flexibility, endurance, coordination, and proprioception are the goals of these workouts. As a patient's health improves, therapists create exercise regimens that are customized to the patient's unique demands and goals, progressively increasing in complexity and intensity.

Exercises for Range of Motion:

The goal of range of motion (ROM) exercises is to increase the range of motion and flexibility in the elbow, shoulder, wrist, and hand joints. These exercises can involve joint mobilizations and stretching methods in addition to passive, active-assisted, and active range of motion exercises. Restoring normal joint motion and avoiding contractures or stiffness are the objectives.

Strengthening Activities:

Strengthening exercises improve muscle power, endurance, and functional capacity by focusing on the hand, wrist, forearm, and upper arm muscles. Exercises with resistance bands, free weights, therapeutic putty, or specialized equipment are prescribed by therapists to gradually challenge the muscles while preserving correct form and alignment.

Reflexology Training:

The body's capacity to perceive its limbs' orientation, movement, and position in space is known as proprioception. Enhancing proprioception and neuromuscular control in the hand and upper extremities is the main goal of proprioceptive training exercises. Proprioceptive feedback devices, balance drills, and functional activities that test stability and coordination are a few examples of these workouts.

Techniques for Scar Management:

Scar tissue can develop after trauma or surgery and impair hand and upper extremity movement and function. The goals of scar management procedures are to maximize tissue healing, reduce adhesions, and enhance scar flexibility. These methods could involve silicone gel sheets, compression therapy, scar massage, stretching, and modalities including laser or ultrasound therapy.

Training in Activities of Daily Living (ADL):

The goal of ADL training is to increase a person's capacity to carry out necessary daily chores safely and independently. When necessary, therapists employ adapted techniques and equipment to mimic daily tasks like feeding, dressing, grooming, cooking, and cleaning the house. ADL instruction improves a person's quality of life and fosters functional independence.

Practical Instruction:

Functional training entails performing particular motions or tasks that are pertinent to a person's personal, professional, and leisure pursuits. Based on the goals and functional impairments of the individual, therapists create functional training programs that enhance skill acquisition and performance through task-specific exercises and simulated work or leisure activities.

Therapists can address the special needs and difficulties of people with hand and upper extremity injuries, surgeries, or conditions by incorporating these treatment approaches into an all-encompassing rehabilitation program. This will enable the patients to achieve the best possible recovery, functional independence, and participation in meaningful activities.

Rehabilitation Modalities

In order to control pain, encourage tissue repair, and enhance function, modalities are therapeutic instruments and approaches used in rehabilitation. The following modalities are frequently employed in hand and upper extremity rehabilitation:

Both Cryotherapy and Heat Therapy:

Heat Therapy: Using heat treatments like paraffin baths or wet heat packs can help reduce pain and stiffness by relaxing muscles and increasing blood flow. To increase tissue extensibility and make stretching easier, heat therapy is frequently utilized prior to manual therapy or therapeutic exercises.

Cryotherapy: By narrowing blood vessels and numbing the affected area, cold treatments like ice packs or cold compresses can help lessen pain, edema, and inflammation. After physical therapy or exercise, cryotherapy is frequently used to reduce post-exercise soreness and manage discomfort.

Electrical Induction:

Transcutaneous Electrical Nerve Stimulation (TENS): TENS machines use electrodes applied to the skin to administer low-voltage electrical impulses that block pain signals to the brain and encourage the release of endorphins, which are the body's natural analgesics.

Neuromuscular Electrical Stimulation (NMES): NMES is the application of electrical stimulation to muscles in order to enhance strength, cause contractions, and avoid atrophy, especially in those who are paralyzed or have weakness as a result of nerve injury or lack of use.

Therapy with Ultrasound:

High-frequency sound waves are used in ultrasound therapy to produce deep tissue heating, which can speed up the healing process, encourage tissue relaxation, and boost blood flow. Because ultrasound enhances tissue flexibility and reduces pain and inflammation, it is frequently used to treat soft tissue injuries, such as tendonitis or ligament sprains.

Taping Methods:

Applying kinesiology tape to the skin can offer pain relief, support, and stability without limiting mobility. It can lessen edema, increase proprioception, and assist muscles work better when engaging in certain activities.

Rigid Taping: During sports or rehabilitation, rigid tape is used to support or immobilize joints to provide stability and prevent overuse or damage.

Splinting and Assistive Technology:

Assistive Devices: People with hand and upper extremity disabilities can benefit from a variety of assistive devices, including reachers, dressing aids, ergonomic tools, and adaptive utensils, to help them carry out everyday chores safely and freely.

Splinting: Injured or surgically repaired joints, tendons, or ligaments are frequently immobilized, supported, or shielded using customized splints or orthotic devices. During the recovery phase, splints can also lessen pain, support functional tasks, and help preserve normal alignment.

These modalities are frequently combined with manual therapy, therapeutic exercises, and other rehabilitation strategies to help people with ailments, surgeries, and injuries involving the hands and upper extremities recover as quickly as possible. Therapists choose and adapt modalities with great care, taking into account each patient's unique needs, preferences, and therapy objectives.

CHAPTER FIVE
Therapeutic Interventions for Specific Conditions

Of course! An outline of therapy approaches for particular ailments affecting the hand and upper limb is provided below:

Recovery after Breaks:

Immobilization: In order to preserve the bones and encourage healing, the fractured area may first be immobilized with splints, casts, or braces.

activities for Range of Motion: To avoid stiffness and preserve joint mobility when the fracture starts to heal, mild activities for range of motion should be started.

Progressive Strengthening: To restore muscle strength and endurance as the healing process advances, progressive strengthening activities are included.

Functional Training: To encourage the return of functional independence, functional tasks and activities that are applicable to the person's everyday life are included.

Treatment for Arthritis:

Pain Management: To control pain and inflammation, techniques including heat therapy, cold packs, or transcutaneous electrical nerve stimulation (TENS) can be applied.

Exercises for Range of Motion: Mild stretches and range-of-motion drills assist in preserving joint flexibility and lowering stiffness.

Strengthening Exercises: To improve support and stability for the afflicted joints, strengthening exercises concentrate on strengthening the surrounding muscles.

Joint Protection strategies: People can reduce the amount of stress placed on their arthritic joints during daily activities by learning about ergonomics and joint protection strategies.

Treatment for Bursitis and Tendinitis:

Activity Modification: You can lessen the strain on the injured tendons or bursae by avoiding activities that make your symptoms worse and by using different strategies.

Modalities: To lessen pain and inflammation, electrical stimulation, ultrasound, or ice therapy may be applied.

Stretching and Strengthening: To increase flexibility, strength, and endurance, specific stretching and strengthening activities are performed on the impacted muscles and tendons.

Gradual Return to Activities: Resuming sports and activities gradually while keeping an eye on symptoms aids in long-term healing and helps avoid recurrence.

Rehabilitating Nerve Damage:

Sensory Reeducation: Regaining sensation and enhancing proprioception in the affected area are achieved through the use of sensory reeducation procedures.

Motor Re-education: Through specific workouts and activities, motor re-education exercises aim to restore muscle strength, coordination, and function.

Exercises for Nerve Gliding: These exercises facilitate nerve mobilization and guard against adhesions or entrapment when moving.

Functional Training: To increase hand dexterity and functional independence, functional tasks and exercises are included.

Handling Carpal Tunnel Syndrome Rehabilitation:

Splinting: To maintain the wrist in a neutral position and relieve pressure on the median nerve, wear wrist splints at night.

Gentle nerve gliding exercises are a good way to release tension and mobilize the median nerve.

Stretching and Strengthening: Both stretching and strengthening exercises serve to increase the flexibility and balance of the hand and forearm muscles.

Activity Modification: Making ergonomic changes and adaptations to routine tasks might assist lessen wrist strain from repetitive motion.

Trigger finger rehabilitation:

Splinting: Resting the tendon and lowering triggering are achieved by splinting the injured finger in a straight position.

Exercises for Tendon Gliding: These exercises aid in reducing adhesions and enhancing tendon mobility.

Modalities: Ultrasound or heat therapy are two options for treating stiffness and pain.

Activity Modification: Repetitive grabbing and gripping activities should be avoided in order to reduce symptoms and avoid aggravating them.

In order to treat Dupuytren's contracture:

Splinting: To gradually extend and straighten the afflicted fingers, dynamic or night splinting may be utilized.

Manual Therapy: Myofascial release and massage are examples of manual methods that can assist enhance finger mobility and lessen tension in the tissues.

Stretching and Strengthening: To preserve flexibility and stop the return of contractures, perform hand and finger stretching and strengthening exercises.

Surgical Intervention: To restore finger function in extreme situations, a surgical release of the contracture may be required.

Amputation Rehabilitation:

Prosthetic Training: After having an upper limb amputated, individuals receive training on how to operate and maintain prosthetic equipment.

Desensitization techniques: People can better tolerate prosthetics and adjust to changes in feeling with the use of desensitization exercises and sensory re-education.

Training for Strength and Coordination: The goal of strengthening exercises and functional activities is to increase the strength and coordination of the residual limbs.

Psychological Support: To assist people in overcoming the emotional and psychological difficulties brought on by limb loss, counseling and support groups are offered.

The goal of rehabilitation for certain conditions is to meet each person's special needs and obstacles in order to maximize healing, promote functional independence, and enhance quality of life. Physical therapists, occupational therapists, and other medical specialists are included in multidisciplinary treatment regimens that are customized to each patient's condition, goals, and preferences.

Psychological Considerations in Rehabilitation

Psychological factors are essential to the rehabilitation process because they help people deal with pain, impairment, and the difficulties of healing. The following are some essential elements of psychological factors in rehabilitation:

Handling Pain and Incapacity:

Pain Management Techniques: During rehabilitation, people can better control their pain and discomfort by learning about pain management techniques such as deep breathing exercises, relaxation techniques, and cognitive-behavioral tactics.

Psychological Support: To manage the psychological effects of pain, disability, and loss of function, counseling, support groups, and individual therapy sessions offer coping mechanisms and emotional support.

Acceptance and Adaptation: Helping people accept the limits placed on them by an accident or disability and supporting flexible coping mechanisms enable them to adapt to their new situation and concentrate on attainable objectives.

The Value of Education for Patients

Knowing the Situation: Giving patients accurate information about their diagnosis, course of treatment, and alternatives for care gives them the power to take an active role in their recovery and make decisions about their care.

Self-Management Skills: By teaching people how to take charge of their health and effectively manage their condition outside of treatment sessions, we may help them learn self-care practices, at-home exercise regimens, activity moderation, and adaptive methods.

Assisting patients in establishing reasonable expectations for their recuperation process, taking into account possible obstacles and disappointments, promotes positivity and adaptability.

Drive and Involvement:

Establishing relevant and attainable short- and long-term goals together encourages people to be involved in their rehabilitation and to keep their attention on their advancement.

Positive Reinforcement: Giving compliments, encouragement, and positive feedback for accomplishments and advancements increases self-esteem and motivation.

Intrinsic Motivation: Long-term commitment to the rehabilitation process is fostered by highlighting the individual advantages and values of rehabilitation, such as increased independence, quality of life, and engagement in meaningful activities.

Overcoming Psychological Obstacles:

Fear Avoidance: Cognitive-behavioral therapies that address fear avoidance behaviors and negative views about pain and movement assist people in overcoming obstacles to development and increasing their engagement in rehabilitation activities.

Depression and Anxiety: Treating the psychological effects of chronic pain, disability, or catastrophic injury requires screening for signs of depression and anxiety, offering suitable psychological interventions, or referring patients to mental health specialists.

Healthcare providers can assist patients in surmounting obstacles to recovery, fostering adaptability, and augmenting their general state of well-being by attending to psychological aspects of rehabilitation. Optimizing results and fostering long-term success require a comprehensive strategy that incorporates the social, psychological, and medical facets of treatment.

CHAPTER SIX
Recovery and Long-Term Management

Returning to work and regular activities after rehabilitation entails reducing the chance of re-injury or symptom exacerbation while promoting recovery and long-term management. Here are some crucial things to remember:

Going Back to Work and Other Activities:

Gradual Return: People can develop tolerance and confidence while keeping an eye on their symptoms and functional abilities by progressively returning job assignments and daily activities.

Activity Pacing: By encouraging people to pace themselves and take regular breaks during their activities, we can lower the likelihood of flare-ups by preventing overexertion and weariness.

Activity Modification: To ensure safe participation and reduce the risk of worsening symptoms, job tasks or leisure activities can be modified to accommodate physical restrictions or functional impairments.

Strategies for Work Modification:

Ergonomic Assessment: Identifying possible risk factors for musculoskeletal injuries and putting ergonomic improvements into practice are facilitated by doing ergonomic assessments of workstations and occupational tasks.

Redesigning a profession to lessen physical demands or repetitive motions might assist accommodate functional limitations and prevent injuries from overuse.

Assistive Technology: People can work more comfortably and productively when they have access to assistive technology, such as ergonomic tools, adaptive equipment, or employment adjustments.

Modifiable Tools and Methods: The employment of assistive devices, such as dressing aids, reachers, ergonomic keyboards, or adaptable utensils, can alleviate strain on the hands and upper extremities during routine tasks.

Orthotic Devices: Individuals can participate in activities with more comfort and stability while wearing custom splints or orthotic devices, which support and shield joints, tendons, or ligaments.

Adaptive Techniques: Providing alternative movement patterns and adaptive techniques to individuals can help them keep their independence and make up for functional deficiencies.

The Value of Ergonomics

Prevention of Musculoskeletal Injuries: By putting ergonomic concepts into practice at work and at home, one can lower the risk of repetitive strain injuries and prevent musculoskeletal injuries.

Enhancement of Work Performance: By mitigating physical discomfort and tiredness, ergonomic modifications such as appropriate workplace arrangement, adequate posture, and neutral joint alignment enhance work performance and productivity.

Improvement of Comfort and Well-Being: Establishing ergonomic settings that support safety, comfort, and well-being improves people's quality of life in general and lowers their risk of chronic pain or impairment.

Through the integration of these methods into rehabilitation and long-term management plans, people can reduce their risk of injury or functional decline and successfully reintegrate into everyday activities and work. Effective intervention implementation and sustained engagement in work and leisure activities require cooperation among healthcare providers, employers, and individuals themselves.

Preventing Re-injury

Combining techniques to maintain strength, flexibility, and appropriate biomechanics is necessary to prevent re-injury and to preserve long-term health and function in the hand and upper extremities. Here are some proactive measures people can take to avoid getting hurt again:

Sustaining Power and Adaptability:

Frequent Exercise: To preserve muscular strength and joint

mobility in the hand, wrist, forearm, and upper arm, perform strength and flexibility exercises on a frequent basis.

A balanced workout program should include a range of workouts that target various muscle groups to guarantee that the upper extremities are generally strong and stable.

Progressive Overload: To continuously test and enhance muscle strength and endurance, progressively increase the duration, resistance, and intensity of exercises over time.

The right body mechanics

Posture Awareness: To lessen stress on the spine, shoulders, and upper extremities, maintain proper posture while going about your daily business, at work, and during leisure activities.

Lifting Techniques: To reduce strain on the upper body, use proper lifting techniques, such as bending at the knees and lifting using the legs rather than the back.

Joint protection: Steer clear of uncomfortable postures that are repeated or maintained since these can put stress on the hand and upper extremity joints. To lessen strain on the hands and wrists when performing jobs, use ergonomic tools and adaptable equipment.

Paying Attention to Your Body:

Pain Awareness: During activities, be alert for any warning indications of pain, discomfort, or exhaustion. When necessary, take breaks, and change jobs or hobbies that make symptoms worse.

Rest and Recovery: To avoid overuse injuries and encourage tissue repair, make sure you schedule enough time for rest and recovery in between workouts or activities.

Seek Professional Advice: If you're having chronic or getting worse symptoms, it's advisable to speak with a healthcare provider. Timely treatment and early intervention can help prevent more injuries.

Factors related to lifestyle:

Healthy Lifestyle Options: To promote general musculoskeletal health and recovery, choose a healthy lifestyle that includes frequent exercise, a balanced diet, enough hydration, and enough sleep.

Stress management: To ease tension and encourage relaxation in the upper body, engage in stress-reduction practices like mindfulness training, relaxation exercises, or meditation.

Strategies for Preventing Injuries:

Warm-up and Cool-down: To prepare the muscles and joints for movement and aid in recovery, give priority to warm-up exercises prior to physical activity and cool-down stretches afterwards.

Appropriate Equipment Use: To reduce the risk of harm, wear ergonomic and safety gear when playing sports and having fun.

Cross-training: To avoid overuse injuries and preserve general function and fitness, mix up your routine with different workouts and activities.

People can lower their chance of re-injury, preserve their ideal level of strength and flexibility, and support the long-term health and function of their hands and upper extremities by putting these preventive measures into practice and paying attention to their bodies' signals.

THE END

www.ingramcontent.com/pod-product-compliance
Lightning Source LLC
Chambersburg PA
CBHW070315230526
45470CB00002B/881